Dr. S⌐ⅎᵢ

Cure and Recipes

The Complete Guide to Cure Diseases,

Detox Your Body and Lose Weight

with Natural Remedies

Hanna Miller

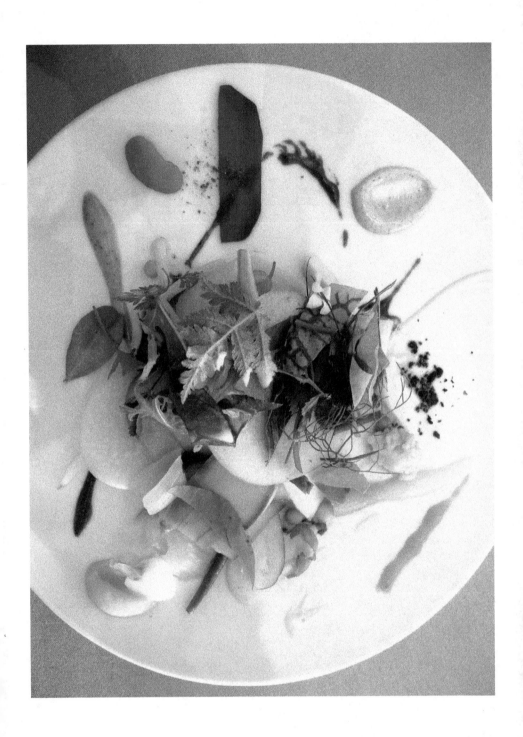

Table of Contents

Introduction

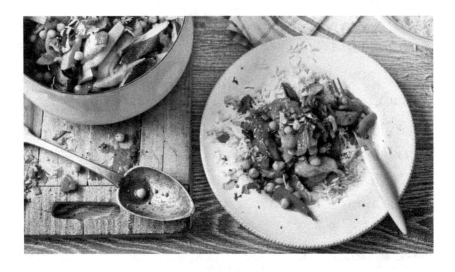

The Alkaline Diet and Intracellular Cleansing

The Alkaline Diet is a way of eating that balances your pH levels by choosing the right foods, mostly alkaline based, to maintain good health. Becoming familiar with the right types of food items to include in your diet is as simple as learning whether each item on your grocery list is alkaline or acidic.

Before your next trip to the supermarket, review the list of items or write down the foods you usually include on a typical shopping trip. For example, your list may contain the following items:

- Milk (2L)

- Bread

- Yogurt

- Apples (1 bag)

- Butter

- Ground beef (2 lbs.)

- Breakfast sausage

- Potatoes (1 bag)

- Eggs (1 dozen)

- Spinach (frozen)

- Case of pop/soda (12 cans)

- Tomatoes

- Mayonnaise

- Granola bars (1 box)

- Garlic

In total, there are fifteen items on this grocery list. How many of them are acidic versus alkaline? The results may be surprising:

<u>Acidic:</u> milk, bread, yogurt, butter, ground beef, breakfast sausage, eggs, pop/soda, mayonnaise, granola bars

<u>Alkaline:</u> apples, potatoes, spinach, tomatoes, garlic

Two-thirds of these items are acidic, while the remaining is alkaline. It is important to note that all the alkaline foods on this list are vegetables and fruits. In general, nearly all fruits and vegetables are alkaline-based, which makes a plant-based diet a good foundation to build an alkaline diet. The key is a balance, even with acidic foods as part of your regular diet, by increasing the alkaline content significantly over time. This will have a major improvement in your health in many ways.

Below is an idea of how your shopping list might look if you choose to follow Dr. Sebi's diet.

Fruit

Add any of the following Dr. Sebi-approved fruits to your shopping list:

- Bananas
- Apples
- Currants
- Berries
- Cantaloupe
- Dates

- Figs

- Tamarind

- Papayas

- Oranges

- Pears

- Plums

- Melons

- Peaches

- Cherries

- Grapes

- Limes

- Mangoes

- Raisins

- Prunes

Grains

Add any of the following Dr. Sebi-approved grains to your shopping list:

- Wild rice

- Kamut

- Amaranth

- Spelt

- Rye

- Quinoa

- Tef

- Fonio

Vegetables

Add any of the following Dr. Sebi-approved vegetables to your shopping list

- Bell peppers

- Amaranth

- Avocados

- Arame

- Dandelion greens

- Nori

- Lettuce (excluding iceberg)

- Mushrooms

- Garbanzo beans

- Kale

- Chayote

- Onions

- Tomatillo

- Olives

- Okra
- Squash
- Wild arugula
- Zucchini
- Wakame
- Watercress

Excess Mucus in the Body

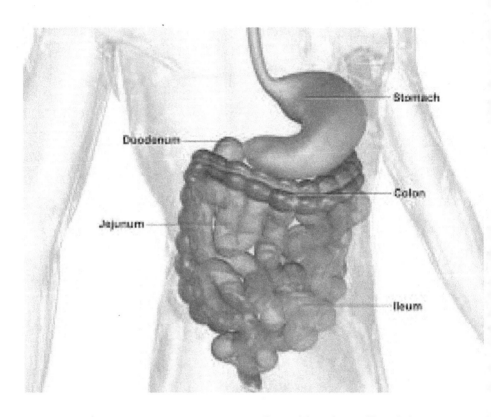

Mucus is an aqueous secretion produced by the cells of the mucous glands. It serves as a covering for the mucous membranes. Mucus is mainly composed of water, which is the mucin secretion.

It is an important element of the epithelial lining fluid, the airway surface liquid, which is the lining of the respiratory tract. Mucus helps to protect the lungs during breathing by trapping foreign particles and infectious agents like dust, allergens, virus, bacteria, etc.

The human body always tends to produce more mucus in order to protect and prevent the airway tissues from drying out. Thus, there is a continuous production of mucus in the respiratory system.

When foreign objects get trapped by the mucus, the mucus becomes thick and changes color most of the time. This thick mucus that is usually coughed out as sputum is known as phlegm.

Mucus also plays an important role in the digestive system. The layer formed by the mucus in the small intestine and colon helps to protect the intestinal epithelial cells from bacterial infections. It also serves as a lubricant for the movement of foods through the esophagus.

Interestingly, mucus is the body's natural lubricant in females which helps during sexual intercourse. It also helps to fight against infection in the reproductive system.

Mucus and the Health of the Body

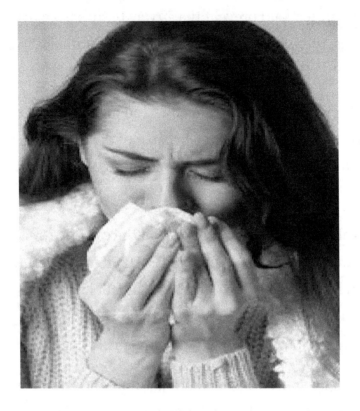

There is a continuous process of mucus production in the body, which helps to protect the body systems from infections and also provides necessary lubrication to the body.

Thus, the presence of mucus in our bodies is important. When mucus traps foreign and infectious bodies, it becomes phlegm. Phlegm and excess mucus in the body is not healthy. As the body produces up to a liter of mucus every day, it is vital to get rid of it to keep the body healthy.

Accumulation of mucus in the body is the major cause of illnesses as claimed by Dr. Sebi. So, excess mucus can be a red flag for an unhealthy state of the body.

Causes of Mucus Buildup in the Body

Just like in snails and other animals that secrete mucus, there are triggers for the production of mucus. In human beings, the major triggers are dryness and inflammation of the body. Some factors that may lead to dryness, inflammation, and other mucus secretion triggers are:

- Dry air

- Smoking

- Allergies

- Infections

- Acid reflux

- Asthma

- Low water/liquid consumption

- Medications etc.

These factors and more contribute to excess buildup of mucus in the body. The body naturally produces mucus to ensure that foreign objects (toxic and/or infectious) don't interact with the body cells. The more we have these foreign bodies, the more the body produces mucus.

When these objects get trapped by the mucus, the mucus becomes thick and builds up as phlegm.

Moreover, our body must stay lubricated for the swift movement of particles and cells in the body. Thus, dryness of the body makes the body produce more mucus, which is the liquid the body can produce naturally.

Electric Food - Acid and Alkaline

Some foods and drinks change from acidic to alkaline once they are metabolized. This essentially makes them alkaline based, as once they are digested, they become alkaline. One of the most common foods in this category is citrus fruits, which contain ascorbic acid.

Citrus Fruits

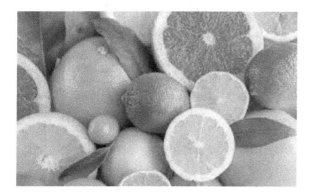

Citrus fruits may be often avoided as they are often considered acidic and sour to taste. Once they are fully digested, they effectively become alkaline in the body, with the results of increasing the pH balance to a more basic or alkaline environment. Fruits that fit into this category include lime, lemon, oranges, mandarins, tangerines, and grapefruit.

Tomatoes

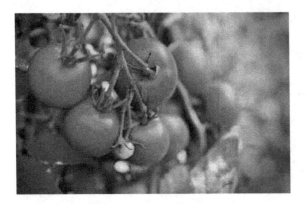

Tomatoes are another example of a fruit that becomes rich in alkaline once consumed. They are naturally acidic, and like citrus fruits, may be avoided due to their sour and sometimes strong taste. Tomatoes are best consumed in a raw state when they are digested quickly and increase the alkaline levels in the blood. When they are stewed, baked, or otherwise cooked, tomatoes increase in acidity, though are still very nutritious. If you enjoy tomatoes or cooked varieties are a regular part of your diet, incorporate both raw and cooked versions. For example, if you create pasta dishes, stew some tomatoes, and add some raw slices or cherry tomatoes as a topping to gain their benefits.

Kombucha Drinks

Kombucha is an acidic beverage that is comprised of fermented ingredients. It is typically created with a tea base (green or black tea), with added sugar for the fermentation process to form healthy bacterial cultures. There are many varieties of kombucha and recipes for flavoring and fermentation techniques. Kombucha drinks are growing in popularity in grocery stores and restaurants, though they were once considered a rare treat in upscale eateries and shops. They are available in many flavors and contain a longer shelf life than other fermented foods, such as yogurt, kimchi, and sauerkraut.

Why is kombucha beneficial for an alkaline diet? Although it is an acidic beverage, once metabolized, it becomes alkaline in the body. It is beneficial for gut health and aiding in the digestion process, which is due to the role of healthy bacteria, which also prevents infectious diseases and conditions, many of which originate in the gut. The healthy bacteria act as a barrier or protection in the stomach during the digestion process, which keeps acidic levels low to moderate. Kombucha is also high in antioxidants, which is a good defense against cancer, diabetes, and other conditions (for treatment and prevention), which is why this drink is beneficial as part of an alkaline diet.

Pineapples

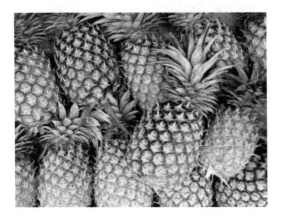

Many people will avoid pineapples because they can taste sour and cause irritation initially, though they are high in nutrients and alkalinize in the body once consumed. The benefits of pineapples include improving gut health, similarly, to fermented foods, such as yogurt and kombucha. Pineapples also reduce bloating and inflammation, which is caused by a lot of chronic and autoimmune conditions. Joint pain, arthritis, and other conditions that impact the bones and joints can be improved by the high amount of vitamin C and antioxidants in pineapples. Vitamin C improves the immunity function, which is beneficial for good health in general. If you exercise regularly and include weight or powerlifting as a part of your workout, eating pineapples and fruits high in vitamin C, fiber, and alkaline (once digested) can help your muscles recover quickly.

Apple Cider Vinegar

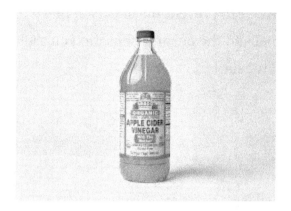

There are a lot of reported health benefits of adding apple cider vinegar to your diet, even in small amounts such as a tablespoon or two each day. This is made by mixing fermented apples with yeast and bacteria. Due to the acetic acid levels contained in it, many people avoid it altogether, as it has a pungent taste that is difficult to swallow. Diluting with water or lemon juice is one way to offset the strong taste, as well as adding to a balsamic dressing or another condiment. The benefits of apple cider vinegar work well with an alkaline diet for the following reasons:

Apple cider vinegar benefits insulin sensitivity and keeps blood sugar levels normal. While not conclusive, this effect may decrease the likelihood of developing type 2 diabetes.

Taken after a meal, it can help with the digestive process and curb overeating, which can promote weight loss and management.

It's best to consume with water or diluted with a similar drink such as tea or sparkling water to prevent the effects of the acetic acid on tooth enamel and the burning sensation on the mouth and throat if used regularly.

Hot Peppers (Including Cayenne Pepper)

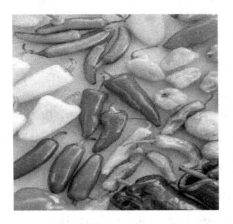

Peppers, the hot and spicy variety, and cayenne pepper, in particular, can provide a lot of health benefits. Most peppers are acidic naturally; though contain a lot of vitamin C and other nutrients that are good for your body. Cayenne pepper, specifically, becomes alkaline once it is ingested, which is a great reason to use as a seasoning in your meals, especially if you have a spicy palate. Most varieties of cayenne pepper are available in a dried, powder form, which makes it easy to use and extends the shelf life. The most important benefits of this spice are as follows:

When your body experiences pain, such as a headache or backache, cayenne provides a way of stimulating the body's response system in such a way that it diverts the sensation from the nerves, therefore decreasing the feeling of pain. In some natural remedies, cayenne is used as an ingredient to treat joint and muscle pain as a topical cream or oil.

There are some indications that cayenne pepper may aid with metabolism, which has a positive impact on weight loss. When your body produces heat, this increases the metabolism process. Cayenne pepper assists with this process, especially when enjoyed as part of a regular meal plan. While studies show that cayenne may not have consistent results in increasing metabolism over some time, it's important to note the initial benefit, as this can be a good way to start a weight loss plan.

Cayenne may suppress hunger, making you feel fuller faster and delaying the next meal or portion size. To make the most of this benefit, some people choose to take cayenne in a supplement form, such as capsules, which can usually be found in a natural health food store. If this is a supplement you want to include in your daily routine, consider finding the most natural, organic option available to ensure the maximum amount of benefits.

A lot of autoimmune conditions can be improved by changing diet, by alleviating symptoms to impact the underlying cause of the condition directly. One such condition is psoriasis, which is often treated with medications and topical creams.

Capsaicin is an ingredient in cayenne, and as with creams for the treatment of joint and related pain relief, this ingredient is also used for psoriasis. Long-term benefits of reducing or possibly eliminating psoriasis by inhibiting the production of substance P in the body, which is primarily responsible for creating this condition.

Cayenne pepper is high in vitamin C and antioxidants, which can prevent and slow cancerous cell growth. Prostate, skin, and pancreatic cancers are among the types that can be prevented by cayenne pepper's nutritional ingredients.

The best benefit of cayenne pepper is how easy it is to add to most meals to enhance flavor. They are safe to eat and an excellent way to enjoy spicy food.

Roles and Food Principles

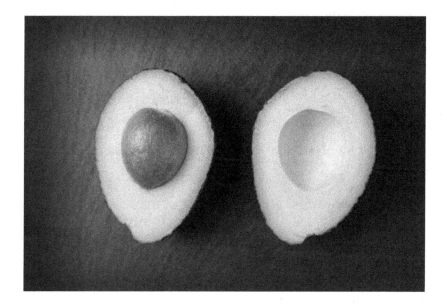

Even if you don't understand how most diets work, you know that processed meats are very bad for you when it comes to health and wellness. There have been many studies showing that processed meat can cause many diseases and illnesses. Moreover, they happen to be backed up with detailed studies to prove as such. When following the alkaline diet, you are not allowed to eat any processed meat. It makes this diet one of the better diets when it comes to living a healthier life. Given all the benefits, you can now see how it can be an excellent idea for you to start following this diet.

Which is why they face more adversities when it comes to diseases in those specific areas; If you live in North America or a European country, then you will be facing a lot more of these diseases and problems. One of the most important things when it comes to eating processed meat is that it has been linked to an unhealthy lifestyle. Processed meat has been associated with being around people who are living an unhealthy life overall. Also, as you know, many people in the United States tend to live an unhealthy lifestyle and eat a ton of processed food. One example would be that many people who smoke cigarettes tend to eat a lot of processed meats.

Also, people who drink much alcohol will consume a lot of processed meat when they are intoxicated. This is a prevalent practice, which makes it a very unhealthy lifestyle decision. Ask yourself, when was the last time you consumed processed meat, there is a high chance that you were intoxicated the last time you consumed processed meat. Most of the time, you are eating processed meats when you are intoxicated or smoking a lot of cigarettes; moreover, people who eat a lot of processed meat tend to consume fewer fruits and vegetables.

If you're not eating the right amount of fiber and micronutrients in your diet, then there's a high chance that you're not living a healthy life overall. Basically, people who are not living a healthy life tend to consume a lot of processed meats. If you're one of them, then make sure that you rectify this situation as quickly as possible by cutting out the unhealthy things in your life which includes processed meat. Another thing that processed meat has been linked with would be chronic diseases. Eating processed meat can increase the risk of high blood pressure, heart diseases, cancer, and chronic obstructive pulmonary disease. There have been many studies showings, the people who eat this kind of meat tend to have a higher chance of attracting diseases stated above. There have also been studies done on an animal that has been consuming processed meat, and it showed that their cancer risk where bought higher when consuming processed meat as compared to when there were not.

The reason why is because processed meat contains harmful chemicals that may increase the risk of chronic diseases. There are numerous chemicals in processed meat; one of them is nitrite. This compound is one of the main reasons why your risk of cancer increases when consuming processed meat. This is the reason why the use of the compound is to preserve the red, pink color of the meat. It also helps to improve the taste of the meat and finally to get rid of any bacteria or growth in the long-term. Another reason why processed meat cannot be right for you is that it has been smoked. As we know, meat smoking is widespread when it comes to preservation.

It has often been salted and dried, to extend the shelf life of it. Once you get meat smoked in a burning wood and charcoal with dripping fat burns on a hot surface, it can cause many chemicals to form in the heat and hence making the meat very unhealthy. This is why it isn't a good idea to consume processed meats in the long-term, the way it has been made and processed makes it a terrible idea for you to consume it. There was one study done that showed when consuming processed meat every day equals smoking ten cigarettes a day in regard to the health affects you might face when consuming processed meat. This goes to show how bad processed meat can be for you. Another thing is that processed meat contains trans-fat. As you know, trans-fat is a human-made fat which has been causing many side effects on our health and wellness.

A decent amount of good fats in our diet is significant for optimal hormone production, etc. However, trans-fat can be very bad for us in the long term as it can cause many problems. One of the issues you might face when consuming trans-fat is the lowered amount of good cholesterol and the increase of bad cholesterol. Also, processed meat contains a lot of sodium, which can be very bad for us in the long-term. As you know, high amounts of sodium consumption can cause many illnesses and diseases. One of the significant things that it can cause is the risk of high blood pressure. High amounts of sodium have shown to increase blood pressure and inflammation increase, which is why it is not advisable for people to eat a lot of sodium when consuming processed meat. Processed meat can cause a lot of issues as we know by now, but one of the significant things that has been found in recent studies is that there is an increase in breast cancer.

There was one study that showed that when women consumed processed meat such as hot dogs, the risk of breast cancer went up 9%. This isn't high when you think about it, but it could still be avoided. Overall, the risk of type 2 diabetes will go up 19%, and the risk of heart disease while going up to 42% when consuming processed meat. These studies have been backed up by proper scientific studies done in a lab, which goes to show that processed meat cannot be good for health and overall well-being, which is one of the reasons why the alkaline diet does not allow you to eat meat in general, as a meat has been shown to increase the acidic levels in your body. The whole premise behind the alkaline diet is that you are not to consume foods that will raise your acidic level in your body when you have high acidic levels in your body, and there's a high chance for you to consume more bacteria. When there are more bacteria in your body, there's a high chance for you to attract more diseases and illnesses.

When it comes to attracting disease growing in your body, the bacteria like the acidic environment of your body, hence, when your body is sick, you will attract more of those diseases, and it will be more likely for you to grow them when your body is acidic. One of the most acidic things you can consume would be the use of processed meats. As you know, processed meats can cause many issues. If you're looking to follow the alkaline diet and then there's no chance in hell that you're going to be eating any processed meat. Even if you're someone looking to better your health, the first thing you need to do is cut out any processed meats that you think you're going to eat.

We can tell you what you should do and should not do, but as you can tell by the evidence that processed meat is not the answer when it comes to living a healthier life. More often than not, many of your consuming processed meat, and you don't even know it. Did you know that meats that are not organic and have been cut mechanically are also considered processed meats? These meats have been cut in a way that can cause many issues. Unfortunately, our system has made everything unhealthy when it comes to consuming food.

What to Expect from the Detox

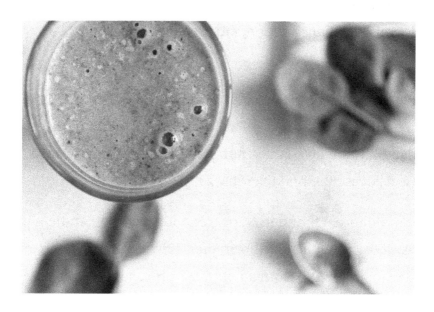

Detoxification is necessary when the body's natural detoxification organs become weak. This occurs as a result of prolonging the impact of stress, illness, poor health habit, improper diet, sedentary lifestyles, overconsumption of foods, exposure to environmental toxic substances, exposure to industrial by-products...and more.

A countless number of the toxic substances are opened to metabolic conversion or deactivation in the body and safely removed out of the body. But, when the body is loaded with environmental chemicals or when its detox organ (Liver) is not functioning well, toxins accumulate in fatty tissues and other body tissues.

Visible symptoms of this accumulation are chronic inflammation, constipation, fatigue, body odor, and overweight.

Some other dangerous effects are suppressed immune function, endocrine, and sexual dysfunction both in males and females, reduced male fertility, diabetes, increased risk for cardiovascular and liver disease.

Some chemicals found in skincare products (like Parabens) are associated with some hormones, accumulate in breast tissue, and excite the spread of human breast cancer cells.

For example, most individual's digestive systems that turn out to be unable to digest food properly; take place as a result of prolonging overconsumption of foods that are high in fats, processed foods, and low fiber foods. When this happens, food cannot move through the digestive tract and produce toxic by-products. This condition is called toxic colon syndrome or intestinal toxemia.

Detoxification is very important for individuals that have chronic health conditions such as Depression, Diabetes, Mental illness, Obesity, Cancer, Digestive disorder, Asthma, Allergies, Anxiety, Headache, High cholesterol, Arthritis, Low blood sugar level, Heart problems, Chronic fatigue syndrome, Fibromyalgia...and many others.

Detoxification is also important for individuals whose health problems are initiated by environmental conditions and for those suffering from allergies and immune deficiency issues that orthodox medicine cannot manage.

What Are the Phases of Detoxification?

As you undergo the process of detoxification, there are three major phases your body will encounter in order to achieve an accurate cure. These phases are:

Purification: in this process, you are expected to take in diets that are readily capable of detoxifying your body. This means that the diets you have to take in should be composed of detoxifying components. In this phase, you should endeavor to eat foods that are healthy and not unhealthy diets.

Restructuring/ reformation: at this phase, the body begins to adjust itself and encourages reformation. The whole system brings itself together to become healthy again.

Maintenance of good health: at this phase, the whole system interprets the information provided during the reformation phase and utilizes it to become perpetually healthy.

What Are the Benefits of Detoxification?

There are bundles of benefits you gain when you undergo the process of detoxification. These benefits are:

- It helps in weight loss and improves the well-being of the body.

- It helps in boosting the energy level.

- It helps in cleaning and strengthening the organs of detoxification and its passageways.

- It helps in boosting fertility in both men and women.

- It helps in improving mental functions.

- It helps in reducing fatigue.

- It helps in improving the appearance of the skin.

- It helps in the improvement of emotional wellbeing.

- It helps in improving memory.

- It helps in the enhancement of skin appearance.

- It helps in alleviating insomnia.

- It reduces the number of toxins in the body.

- It improves the circulatory system.

- It increases the body's immunity.

- It helps in improving optimal concentration.

- It helps in reducing stomach bloating.

- It provides strength for the nails and hair.

- It removes toxins from the liver.

- It helps in the improvement and strengthening of the digestive tract and system.

- It reduces the risk of diseases by improving the urinary system.

Breakfast Recipes

Vegetable Pancakes

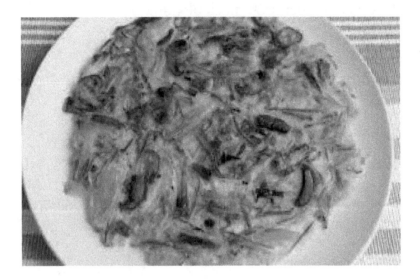

Preparation Time: 5 minutes

Cooking Time: 5 minutes

Serving: 2

Ingredients:

½ white onion, grated

1 yellow squash, roughly chopped

1 zucchini, peeled and chopped

1 zucchini, roughly chopped

½ teaspoon onion powder

¼ cup filtered water, as needed

1 teaspoon salt

¼ cup coconut flour

4 scallions

Directions:

1. Add the yellow squash, zucchini, zucchini, scallions, coconut flour, onion, salt, and onion powder in a food processor. Pulse until blended.

2. Add the water to the mixture to make moist but not runny. The batter will be thick.

3. Spray Pan with cooking spray and heat over medium-high heat.

4. Using an ice-cream scoop to drop batter into the pan. Use a fork to spread your mixture evenly over the pan, pressing down on the pancakes. Brown on both sides of pancakes, cooking for about 5 minutes total.

5. Serve hot and enjoy!

Nutrition: calories 254 fat 12.1 carbs 33.4 protein 6.3

Turnip Bowl

Preparation Time: 5 minutes

Cooking Time: 10 minutes

Serving: 2

Ingredients:

2 turnips, peeled and cubed

1 tablespoon coconut oil

1 red bell pepper, seeded and chopped

1 sweet onion, chopped

¼ cup mushrooms, sliced

4 cups kale

2 chive stalks, chopped

1 teaspoon onion powder

1 teaspoon onion powder

½ teaspoon sea salt

½ teaspoon bouquet garn herb blended, or other dried herbs like sage or rosemary

Directions:

1. In a bowl, combine the turnips, red bell pepper, mushrooms, kale, chives, onion, oil, onion powder, and onion powder.

2. Heat a non-stick cooking pan over medium heat, and cook the vegetables, stirring often for about 10 minutes, or until tender.

3. Serve and Enjoy!

Nutrition: calories 190, fat 2, carbs 18, protein 11

Millet Porridge

Preparation Time: 10 minutes

Cooking Time: 20 minutes

Serving: 2

Ingredients:

Pinch of sea salt

1 tablespoon coconuts, chopped finely

½ cup unsweetened coconut milk

½ cup millet, rinsed and drained

1½ cups water

3 drops liquid stevia

Directions:

1. Sauté millet in a non-stick skillet for 3 minutes. Stir in salt and water. Let it boil then reduce the heat.

2. Cook for 15 minutes then stirs in remaining ingredients. Cook for another 4 minutes.

3. Serve with chopped nuts on top.

Nutrition: calories 219, fat 5, carbs 38, protein 6

Squash Hash

Preparation Time: 2 minutes

Cooking Time: 10 minutes

Serving: 2

Ingredients:

1 teaspoon onion powder

½ cup onion, finely chopped

2 cups spaghetti squash

½ teaspoon sea salt

Directions:

1. Squeeze any extra moisture from spaghetti squash using paper towels. Place the squash into a bowl, then add the onion powder, onion, and salt. Stir to combine.

2. Spray a non-stick cooking skillet with cooking spray and place it over medium heat.

3. Add the spaghetti squash to the pan. Cook the squash for 5 minutes, untouched. Using a spatula, flip the hash browns. Cook for an additional 5 minutes or

until the desired crispness is reached. Serve and Enjoy!

Nutrition: calories 212, fat 6, carbs 10, protein 10

Hemp Seed Porridge

Preparation Time: 5 minutes

Cooking Time: 5 minutes

Serving: 6

Ingredients:

Hemp seed

Stevia

Coconut milk

Directions:

1. Combine the rice and coconut milk in a saucepan over medium heat for 5 minutes. Make sure to stir constantly.

2. Remove the pan from the heat and stir in the Stevia.

3. Divide among 6 bowls.

4. Serve and Enjoy!

Nutrition: calories 219, fat 2, carbs 18, protein 7

Smoothies

Pineapple, Banana & Spinach Smoothie

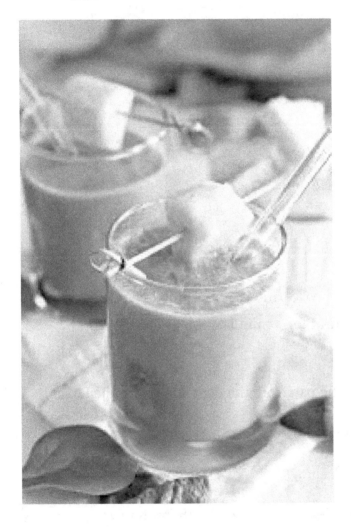

Preparation Time: 10 Minutes

Cooking time: 0 minute

Servings: 1

Ingredients:

½ cup almond milk

¼ cup soy yogurt

1 cup spinach

1 cup banana

1 cup pineapple chunks

1 tbsp. chia seeds

Directions:

1. Add all the ingredients to a blender.

2. Blend until smooth.

3. Chill in the refrigerator before serving.

Nutrition: calories 153, fat 1, carbs 8, protein 1

Spinach Protein Smoothie

Preparation Time: 10 minutes

Cooking Time: 0 minutes

Servings: 2

Ingredients:

1 and 1/2 cups unsweetened coconut milk

1/2 cup yogurt

1/2 teaspoon cinnamon

1 tablespoon protein powder

1/2 banana

2 cups spinach

Directions:

1. Toss in all your ingredients into your blender then process until smooth.

2. Serve and enjoy.

Nutrition: calories 390, fat 1, carbs 24, protein 11

Strawberry Banana Smoothie

Preparation Time: 10 minutes

Cooking Time: 0 minutes

Servings: 1

Ingredients:

1 cup unsweetened coconut milk

1 banana

1/2 cup strawberries

Directions:

1. Add all ingredients to the blender and blend until smooth and creamy.

2. Serve immediately and enjoy.

Nutrition: calories 85, fat 3, carbs 18, protein 11

Easy Mango Lassi

Preparation Time: 10 minutes

Cooking Time: 0 minutes

Servings: 4

Ingredients

2 cups plain whole-milk yogurt

1 cup milk

3 mangoes - peeled, seeded, and chopped

4 tsps. white sugar, or to taste

1/8 tsp. ground cardamom

Directions:

1. In the jar of a blender, place cardamom, white sugar, mangoes, milk, and yogurt.

2. Blend together for about 2 minutes or until smooth.

3. Chill in the refrigerator until cold, about 1 hour.

4. Serve with a small sprinkling of ground cardamom.

Nutrition: calories 220, fat 1, carbs 24, protein 4

Salad and Soups

Coconut Watercress Soup

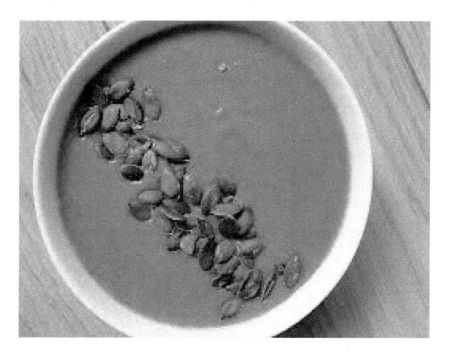

Preparation time: 10 minutes

Cooking time: 20 minutes

Servings: 4

Ingredients:

1 teaspoon coconut oil

1 onion, diced

¾ cup coconut milk

Directions:

1. Preparing the ingredients.

2. Melt the coconut oil in a large pot over medium-high heat. Add the onion and cook until soft, about 5 minutes, then add the peas and the water. Bring to a boil, then lower the heat and add the watercress, mint, salt, and pepper.

3. Cover and simmer for 5 minutes. Stir in the coconut milk and purée the soup until smooth in a blender or with an immersion blender.

4. Try this soup with any other fresh, leafy green— anything from spinach to collard greens to arugula to swiss chard.

Nutrition: calories 170, fat 3, carbs 18, protein 6

Alkaline-Electric Spring Salad

Preparation Time: 11 minutes

Cooking Time: 15 Minutes

Serving: 2

Ingredients

1 cup cherry tomatoes

4 cups seasonal greens

1/4 cup walnuts

1/4 cup approved herbs

For the dressing:

Sea salt and cayenne pepper

3 key limes

1 tablespoon of homemade raw sesame tahini butter

Directions:

1. Sap the key limes.

2. Whisk together the homemade raw sesame "tahini" butter with the key lime juice in a small bowl.

3. Add cayenne pepper and sea salt to your satisfaction.

4. Cut the cherry tomatoes in half.

5. In a large bowl, combine the greens, cherry tomatoes, and herbs. Pour the dressing on top and massage with your hands.

Broccoli Salad Curry Dressing

Preparation Time: 30 Minutes

Cooking Time: 0

Servings: 6

Ingredients:

½ cup plain, unsweetened vegan yogurt

¼ cup onion, chopped

2 heads broccoli florets, chopped

2 stalks celery, chopped

½ teaspoon curry powder

¼ teaspoon salt or to taste

2 tablespoons sunflower seeds

Directions:

1. Mix yogurt, curry powder, and salt.

2. Toss broccoli florets, celery onion, and sunflower seeds.

3. Drizzle the dressing on top and put the salad in the fridge for 30 minutes.

Nutrition: calories 167, fat 1, carbs 18, protein 1

Cherry Tomato Salad with Soy Chorizo

Preparation Time: 5 Minutes

Cooking Time: 5 Minutes

Servings: 4

Ingredients:

2 ½ tbsp. olive oil

4 soy chorizos, chopped

2 tsp. red wine vinegar

1 small red onion, finely chopped

2 ½ cups cherry tomatoes, halved

2 tbsp. chopped cilantro

Salt and freshly ground black pepper to taste

3 tbsp. sliced black olives to garnish

Directions:

1. Heat half a tablespoon of olive oil in a skillet over a medium heat and fry soy chorizo until golden. Turn heat off.

2. In a salad bowl, whisk remaining olive oil and vinegar. Add onion, cilantro, tomatoes, and soy chorizo. Mix with dressing and season with salt and black pepper.

3. Garnish with olives and serve.

Nutrition: calories 130, fat 1, carbs 7, protein 1

Special Ingredients

Homemade Hemp Seed Milk

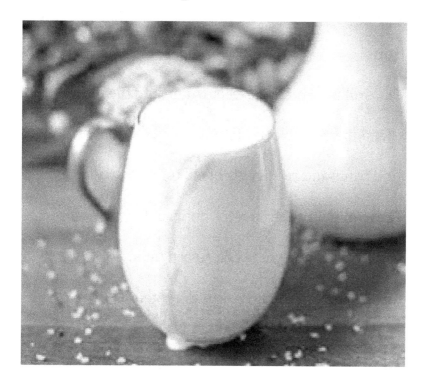

Preparation Time*:* 15 minutes

Cooking Time: 2 hours

Servings*:* 2

Ingredients:

2 tablespoons of hemp seeds

2 tablespoons of agave syrup

1/8 teaspoon of pure sea salt

2 cups of spring water

Fruits (optional)*

Directions:

1. Place all ingredients, except fruits, into the blender.

2. Blend them for two minutes.

3. Add fruits and repeatedly blend for 30 to 50 seconds.

4. Leave milk in a refrigerator until cold.

5. Enjoy your homemade hemp seed milk!

Nutrition: calories 211, fat 1, carbs 8, protein 1

Italian Infused Oil

Preparation Time: 5 minutes

Cooking Time: 24 hours

Servings: 1

Ingredients:

1 teaspoon of oregano

1 teaspoon of basil

1 pinch of pure sea salt

3/4 cup of grapeseed oil

Directions:

1. Fill a glass jar with a lid or a squeeze bottle with grapeseed oil.

2. Mix seasoning together and add them to the jar/bottle.

3. Shake it and let the oil infuse for at least 24 hours.

4. Add it to a dish and enjoy your Italian infused oil!

Nutrition: calories 120, fat 1, carbs 10, protein 1

Garlic Infused Oil

Preparation Time: 5 minutes

Cooking Time: 24 hours

Servings: 1

Ingredients:

1/2 teaspoon of dill

1/2 teaspoon of ginger powder

1 tablespoon of onion powder

1/2 teaspoon of pure sea salt

3/4 cup of grapeseed oil

Directions:

1. Fill a glass jar with a lid or a squeeze bottle with Grape Seed Oil.

2. Add the seasonings to the jar/bottle.

3. Shake it and let the oil infuse for at least 24 hours.

4. Add it to a dish and enjoy your "Garlic" Infused Oil!

Nutrition: calories 130, fat 4, carbs 19, protein 2

Papaya Seed Mango Dressing

Preparation Time: 5 minutes

Cooking Time: 10 minutes

Servings: 2

Ingredients:

1 cup of chopped mango

1 teaspoon of ground papaya seeds

1 teaspoon of basil

1 teaspoon of onion powder

1 teaspoon of agave syrup

2 tablespoons of lime juice

1/4 cup of grapeseed oil

1/4 teaspoon of pure sea salt

Directions:

1. Prepare and place all ingredients into the blender.

2. Blend for one minute until smooth.

3. Add it to a salad and enjoy your papaya seed mango dressing!

Nutrition: calories 320, fat 12, carbs 18, protein 1

Tomato Ginger Dressing

Preparation Time: 5 minutes

Cooking Time: 10 minutes

Servings: 2

Ingredients:

2 chopped plum tomatoes

1 teaspoon of minced ginger*

1 tablespoon of agave syrup

2 tablespoons of chopped onion

2 tablespoons of sesame seeds

1 tablespoon of lime juice

Directions:

1. Prepare and place all ingredients into the blender.

2. Blend for one minute until smooth.

3. Add it to a salad and enjoy your tomato ginger dressing!

Nutrition: calories 1, fat 3, carbs 18, protein 11

Vegetable

Power Pesto Zoodles

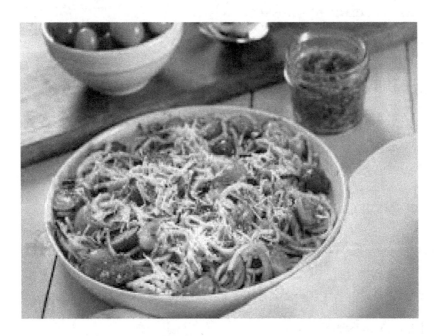

Preparation Time: 10 minutes

Cooking time: 5 minutes

Servings: 2

Ingredients:

2 zucchinis

1 avocado, peeled, pitted

½ cup cherry tomatoes

2 tablespoons walnuts

½ of key lime, juiced

Extra:

¼ teaspoon salt

1/8 teaspoon cayenne pepper

2 teaspoons grapeseed oil

2 tablespoons olive oil

Directions

1. Prepare the zucchini noodles and for this, cut them into thin strips by using a vegetable peeler or use a spiralizer.

2. Then take a medium skillet pan, add oil in it and when hot, add zucchini noodles in it and then cook for 3 to 5 minutes until tender-crisp.

3. Meanwhile, place the remaining ingredients in a food processor and then pulse until the creamy paste comes together.

4. When zucchini noodles have sautéed, drain and place them in a large bowl and add the blended sauce in it.

5. Add 2 tablespoons of water and then toss until well combined.

6. Garnish the zoodles with grated coconut and then serve.

Nutrition: calories 220, fat 11, carbs 18, protein 19

Mushroom Gravy

Preparation Time: 5 minutes

Cooking time: 12 minutes

Servings: 2

Ingredients:

¾ tablespoon spelt flour

¼ of onion, peeled, diced

4 ounces sliced mushrooms

½ cup walnut milk, homemade

1 tablespoon chopped walnuts

Extra:

¼ teaspoon salt

1/8 teaspoon cayenne pepper

½ teaspoon dried thyme

1 tablespoon grapeseed oil

¼ cup vegetable broth, homemade

Directions:

1. Take a medium skillet pan, place it over medium heat, add oil, and when hot, add onion and mushrooms, season with 1/16 teaspoon each of salt and cayenne pepper, and then cook for 4 minutes until tender.

2. Stir in spelt flour until coated, cook for 1 minute, slowly whisk in milk and vegetable broth and then season with remaining salt and cayenne pepper.

3. Switch heat to low-level, cook for 5 to 7 minutes until the sauce has thickened slightly, and then stir in walnuts and thyme.

4. Serve straight away with spelt flour bread.

Nutrition: calories 312, fat 8, carbs 18, protein 10

Nori Burritos

Preparation Time: 10 minutes

Cooking time: 0 minutes

Servings: 2

Ingredients:

1 avocado, peeled, sliced

1 cucumber, deseeded, cut into round slices

1 zucchini, sliced

2 teaspoons sprouted hemp seeds

2 nori sheets

Extra:

1 tablespoon tahini butter

2 teaspoons sesame seeds

Directions:

1. Working on one nori sheet at a time, place it on a cutting board shiny-side-down and then arrange half of each avocado, cucumber and zucchini slices and tahini on it, leaving 1-inch wide spice to the right.

2. Then start folding the sheet over the fillings from the edge that is closest to you, cut into thick slices, and then sprinkle with 1 teaspoon of sesame seeds.

3. Repeat with the remaining nori sheet, and then serve.

Nutrition: calories 210, fat 1, carbs 20, protein 11

Zesty Citrus Salad

Preparation Time: 5 minutes

Cooking time: 0 minutes

Servings: 2

Ingredients:

4 slices of onion

½ of avocado, peeled, pitted, sliced

4 ounces arugula

1 orange, zested, peeled, sliced

1 teaspoon agave syrup

Extra:

1/8 teaspoon salt

1/8 teaspoon cayenne pepper

2 tablespoons key lime juice

2 tablespoons olive oil

Directions:

1. Distribute avocado, oranges, onion, and arugula between two plates.

2. Mix together oil, salt, cayenne pepper, agave syrup, and lime juice in a small bowl and then stir until mixed.

3. Drizzle the dressing over the salad and then serve.

Nutrition: calories 276, fat 3, carbs 18, protein 11

Zucchini Hummus Wrap

Preparation Time: 10 minutes

Cooking time: 8 minutes

Servings: 2

Ingredients:

½ cup iceberg lettuce

1 zucchini, sliced

2 cherry tomatoes, sliced

2 spelt flour tortillas

4 tablespoons homemade hummus

Extra:

¼ teaspoon salt

1/8 teaspoon cayenne pepper

1 tablespoon grapeseed oil

Directions:

1. Take a grill pan, grease it with oil and let it preheat over medium-high heat setting.

2. Meanwhile, place zucchini slices in a large bowl, sprinkle with salt and cayenne pepper, drizzle with oil and then toss until coated.

3. Arrange zucchini slices on the grill pan and then cook for 2 to 3 minutes per side until developed grill marks.

4. Assemble tortillas and for this, heat the tortilla on the grill pan until warm and develop grill marks and spread 2 tablespoons of hummus over each tortilla.

5. Distribute grilled zucchini slices over the tortillas, top with lettuce and tomato slices, and then wrap tightly.

6. Serve straight away.

Nutrition: calories 132, fat 1, carbs 18, protein 10

Dinner Recipes

Roasted Sweet Potatoes

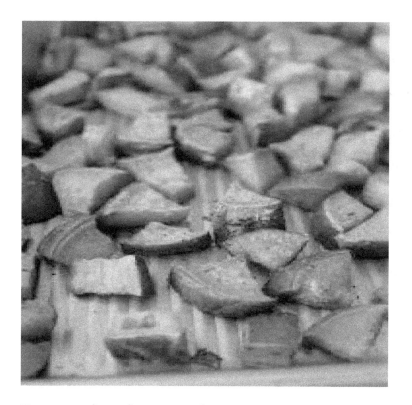

Preparation time: 10 minutes

Cooking time: 45 minutes

Servings: 4

Ingredients:

2 sweet potatoes, peeled and cubed

2½ tablespoons avocado oil

A pinch of salt and black pepper

1 garlic clove, minced

Juice of 1 lime

4 tablespoons water

Directions:

1. Spread the potatoes on a lined baking sheet and combine with the rest of the ingredients.

2. Cook at 400 degrees F for 45 minutes and serve for lunch.

Nutrition: calories 222, fat 6, carbs 15, protein 7

Lemony Carrot Soup

Preparation time: 10 minutes

Cooking time: 40 minutes

Servings: 4

Ingredients:

2 cups carrots, sliced

1 tablespoon olive oil

1 yellow onion, chopped

1½ cups kale, chopped

1 cup plum tomatoes, cubed

3 garlic cloves, minced

A pinch of salt and black pepper

4 teaspoons fresh grated ginger

4 cups water

1 teaspoon sweet paprika

2 teaspoons ground turmeric

Juice of 1 lemon

Zest of ½ lemon, grated

Directions:

1. Heat up a pot with the oil over medium heat, add the onion and garlic, and cook for 5 minutes.

2. Add the carrots and the other ingredients, stir and simmer for 35 minutes more.

3. Divide into bowls and serve.

Nutrition: calories 271, fat 8, carbs 8,3, protein 8

Burrito Bowls

Preparation time: 10 minutes

Cooking time: 0 minutes

Servings: 1

Ingredients:

¼ cup spinach leaves, torn

1 tablespoon chives, chopped

1 tablespoon chopped red bell pepper

1 teaspoon olive oil

3 cherry tomatoes, halved

1 tablespoon chopped parsley

1 red cabbage, shredded

Juice of 1 lime

Directions:

In a bowl, mix the spinach with the chives and the other ingredients, toss, and serve for lunch.

Nutrition: calories 207, fat 3.8, carbs 6, protein 4.4

Mixed Beans Bowls

Preparation time: 10 minutes

Cooking time: 40 minutes

Servings: 4

Ingredients:

1 cup pinto beans, rinsed

1 cup red beans, rinsed

1 cup white beans, rinsed

1 cup soybeans, rinsed

1 yellow onions, chopped

1 tablespoon avocado oil

1 cup cherry tomatoes, halved

1 cup baby spinach

1 small jalapeno pepper, minced

2 teaspoons lime juice

Zest of 1 lime, grated

Salt and black pepper to the taste

1 teaspoon turmeric powder

Directions:

1. Heat up a pan with the oil over medium heat, add the onion, jalapeno and turmeric and cook for 5 minutes.

2. Add the rest of the ingredients, stir and simmer over medium heat for 35 minutes stirring from time to time.

3. Divide into bowls and serve for lunch.

Nutrition: calories 320, fat 12, carbs 12, protein 7

Bell Peppers Soup

Preparation time: 10 minutes

Cooking time: 40 minutes

Servings: 4

Ingredients:

4 shallots, chopped

3 carrots, chopped

1-pound mixed bell peppers, cut into strips

A pinch of salt and black pepper

1 teaspoon hot paprika

4 cups water

1½ cups cauliflower florets, chopped

2 cups kale, chopped

2 tablespoons avocado oil

1 cup cherry tomatoes, chopped

1 teaspoon oregano, dried

Directions:

1. Heat up a pot with the oil over medium-high heat, add the shallots and carrots and cook for 5 minutes.

2. Add the peppers and the other ingredients, stir, simmer over medium heat for 35 minutes more, ladle into bowls and serve for lunch.

Nutrition: calories 210, fat 4.4, carbs 14, protein 6.3

Snacks & Bread

Spinach and Sesame Crackers

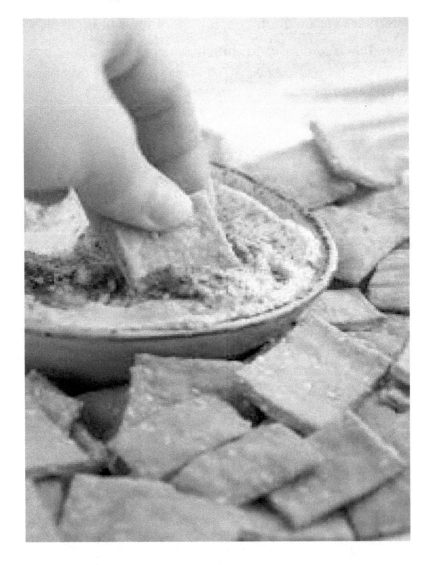

Preparation Time: 5 minutes

Cooking Time: 15 minutes

Servings: 4

Ingredients:

2 tablespoons white sesame seeds

1 cup fresh spinach, washed

1 2/3 cups of all-purpose flour

1/2 cup of water

1/2 teaspoon baking powder

1 teaspoon olive oil

1 teaspoon of salt

Directions:

1. Transfer the spinach to a blender with a half cup of water and blend until smooth.

2. Add 2 tablespoons white sesame seeds, ½ teaspoon baking powder, 1 2/3 cups all-purpose flour, and 1 teaspoon salt to a bowl and stir well until combined. Add in 1 teaspoon olive oil and spinach water. Mix again and knead by using your hands until you obtain a smooth dough.

3. If the made dough is too gluey, then add more flour.

4. Using your parchment paper lightly roll out the dough as thin as possible. Cut into squares with a pizza cutter.

5. Bake in a preheated oven at 400° for about 15to 20 minutes. Once done, let cool and then serve.

Nutrition: calories 190, fat 17, carbs 8, protein 11

Mini Nacho Pizzas

Preparation Time: 5 minutes

Cooking Time: 10 minutes

Servings: 4

Ingredients:

1/4 cup refried beans, vegan

2 tablespoons tomato, diced

2 English muffins, split in half

1/4 cup onion, sliced

1/3 cup vegan cheese, shredded

1 small jalapeno, sliced

1/3 cup roasted tomato salsa

1/2 avocado, diced and tossed in lemon juice

Directions:

1. Add the refried beans/salsa onto the muffin bread.
    Sprinkle with shredded vegan cheese followed by the
    veggie toppings.

2. Transfer to a baking sheet and place in a preheated
    oven at 350 to 400 F on a top rack.

3. Put into the oven for 10 minutes and then broil for 2minutes, so that the top becomes bubbly.

4. Take out from the oven and let them cool at room temperature.

5. Top with avocado. Enjoy!

Nutrition: calories 112, fat 23, carbs 18, protein 28

Pizza Sticks

Preparation Time: 10 minutes

Cooking Time: 30 minutes

Servings: 16 sticks

Ingredients:

5 tablespoons tomato sauce

Few pinches of dried basil

1 block extra firm tofu

2 tablespoon + 2 teaspoon nutritional yeast

Directions:

1. Cape the tofu in a paper tissue and put a cutting board on top, place something heavy on top and drain for about 10 to 15 minutes.

2. In the meantime, line your baking sheet with parchment paper. Cut the tofu into 16 equal pieces and place them on a baking sheet.

3. Spread each pizza stick with a teaspoon of marinara sauce.

4. Sprinkle each stick with a half teaspoon of yeast, followed by basil on top.

5. Bake in a preheated oven at 425 F for about 28 to 30 minutes. Serve and enjoy!

Nutrition: calories 190, fat 23, carbs 8, protein 1

Raw Broccoli Poppers

Preparation Time: 2 minutes

Cooking Time: 8 minutes

Servings: 4

Ingredients:

1/8 cup of water

1/8 teaspoon of fine sea salt

4 cups broccoli florets, washed and cut into 1-inch pieces

1/4 teaspoon turmeric powder

1 cup unsalted cashews, soaked overnight or at least 3-4 hours and drained

1/4 teaspoon onion powder

1 red bell pepper, seeded and

2 heaping tablespoons nutritional

2 tablespoons lemon juice

Directions:

1. Transfer the drained cashews to a high-speed blender and pulse for about 30 seconds. Add in the chopped pepper and pulse again for 30 seconds.

2. Add some 2 tablespoons of lemon juice, 1/8 cup of water, 2 heaping tablespoons of nutritional yeast, ¼ teaspoon of onion powder, 1/8 teaspoon of fine sea salt, and 1/4 teaspoon of turmeric powder. Pulse for about 45 seconds until smooth.

3. Handover the broccoli into a bowl and add in chopped cheesy cashew mixture. Toss well until coated.

4. Transfer the pieces of broccoli to the trays of a yeast dehydrator.

5. Follow the dehydrator's instructions and dehydrate for about 8 minutes at 125 F or until crunchy.

Nutrition: calories 134, fat 18, carbs 6, protein 9

Blueberry Cauliflower

Preparation Time: 2 minutes

Cooking Time: 5 minutes

Servings: 1

Ingredients:

¼ cup of frozen strawberries

2 teaspoons maple syrup

¾ cup unsweetened cashew milk

1 teaspoon vanilla extract

½ cup of plain cashew yogurt

5 tablespoons powdered peanut butter

¾ cup of frozen wild blueberries

½ cup of cauliflower florets, coarsely chopped

Directions:

1. Add all the smoothie ingredients to a high-speed blender.

2. Blitz to combine until smooth.

3. Pour into a chilled glass and serve.

Nutrition: calories 219, fat 11, carbs 8, protein 17

Lunch and Entrées

Green Bean Casserole

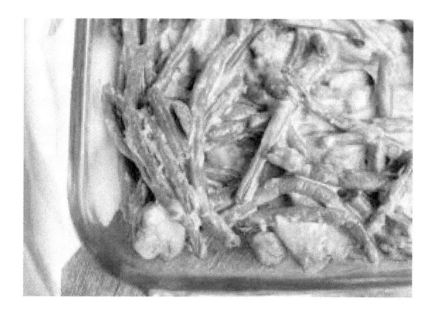

Preparation time: 20 minutes

Cooking Time: 20 minutes.

Servings: 6

Ingredients:

For Onion Slices:

½ cup yellow onion, sliced very thinly

¼ cup almond flour

1/8 tsp garlic powder

Sea salt and freshly ground black pepper, to taste

For Casserole:

1 lb. fresh green beans, trimmed

1 tbsp olive oil

8 oz fresh cremini mushrooms, sliced

½ cup yellow onion, sliced thinly

1/8 tsp garlic powder

Sea salt and freshly ground black pepper, to taste

1 tsp fresh thyme, chopped

½ cup homemade vegetable broth

½ cup coconut cream

Directions:

1. Preheat the oven to 350 degrees F.

2. For onion slices, place all the ingredients in a bowl and toss them to coat the onion well.

3. Arrange the onion slices onto a large baking sheet in a single layer and set it aside.

4. In a pan of salted boiling water, add the green beans and cook for about 5 minutes.

5. Drain the green beans and transfer them into a bowl of ice water.

6. Again, drain well and transfer them again into a large bowl. Set them aside.

7. In a large skillet, heat oil over medium-high heat and sauté the mushrooms, onion, garlic powder, salt, and black pepper for about 2-3 minutes.

8. Stir in the thyme and broth and cook for about 3-5 minutes or until all the liquid is absorbed.

9. Remove from the heat and transfer the mushroom mixture into the bowl with the green beans.

10. Add the coconut cream and stir to combine well.

11. Transfer the mixture into a 10-inch casserole dish.

12. Place the casserole dish and baking sheet of onion slices into the oven.

13. Bake for about 15-17 minutes.

14. Remove the baking dish and sheet from the oven and let it cool for about 5 minutes before serving.

15. Top the casserole with the crispy onion slices evenly.

16. Cut into 6 equal-sized portions and serve.

Nutrition: calories 190, fat 2, carbs 18, protein 32

Vegetarian Pie

Preparation time: 20 minutes

Cooking Time: 1 hour 20 minutes

Servings: 8

Ingredients:

For Topping:

5 cups water

1¼ cups yellow cornmeal

For Filing:

1 tbsp extra-virgin olive oil

1 large onion, chopped

1 medium red bell pepper, seeded and chopped

2 garlic cloves, minced

1 tsp dried oregano, crushed

2 tsp chili powder

2 cups fresh tomatoes, chopped

2½ cups cooked pinto beans

2 cups boiled corn kernels

Directions:

1. Preheat the oven to 375 degrees F. Lightly grease a shallow baking dish.

2. In a pan, add the water over medium-high heat and bring to a boil.

3. Slowly, add the cornmeal, stirring continuously.

4. Reduce the heat to low and cook covered for about 20 minutes, stirring occasionally.

5. Meanwhile, prepare the filling. In a large skillet, heat the oil over medium heat and sauté the onion and bell pepper for about 3-4 minutes.

6. Add the garlic, oregano, and spices and sauté for about 1 minute

7. Add the remaining ingredients and stir to combine.

8. Reduce the heat to low and simmer for about 10-15 minutes, stirring occasionally.

9. Remove from the heat.

10. Place half of the cooked cornmeal into the prepared baking dish evenly.

11. Place the filling mixture over the cornmeal evenly.

12. Place the remaining cornmeal over the filling mixture evenly.

13. Bake for 45-50 minutes or until the top becomes golden brown.

14. Remove the pie from the oven and set it aside for about 5 minutes before serving.

Nutrition: calories 176, fat 1, carbs 10, protein 22

Rice & Lentil Loaf

Preparation time: 20 minutes

Cooking Time: 1 hour 50 minutes

Servings: 8

Ingredients:

1¾ cups plus 2 tbsp filtered water, divided

½ cup wild rice

½ cup brown lentils

Pinch of sea salt

½ tsp no-sodium Italian seasoning

1 medium yellow onion, chopped

1 celery stalk, chopped

6 cremini mushrooms, chopped

4 garlic cloves, minced

¾ cup rolled oats

½ cup pecans, chopped finely

¾ cup homemade tomato sauce

½ tsp red pepper flakes, crushed

1 tsp fresh rosemary, minced

2 tsp fresh thyme, minced

Directions:

1. In a pan, add 1¾ cups of water, rice, lentils, salt, and Italian seasoning and bring them to a boil over medium-high heat.

2. Reduce the heat to low and simmer covered for about 45 minutes.

3. Remove from the heat and set it aside still covered for at least 10 minutes.

4. Preheat the oven to 350 degrees F.

5. With parchment paper, line a 9x5-inch loaf pan.

6. In a skillet, heat the remaining water over medium heat and sauté the onion, celery, mushrooms, and garlic for about 4-5 minutes.

7. Remove from the heat and let it cool slightly.

8. In a large mixing bowl, add the oats, pecans, tomato sauce, and fresh herbs and mix until well combined.

9. Combine the rice mixture and vegetable mixture with the oat mixture and mix well.

10. In a blender, add the mixture and pulse until a chunky mixture forms.

11. Transfer the mixture into the prepared loaf pan evenly.

12. With a piece of foil, cover the loaf pan and bake it for about 40 minutes.

13. Uncover and bake for about 15-20 minutes more or until the top becomes golden brown.

14. Remove it from the oven and set it aside for about 5-10 minutes before slicing.

15. Cut into desired sized slices and serve.

Nutrition: calories 220, fat 3, carbs 8, protein 21

Quinoa & Chickpea Salad

Preparation time: 15 minutes

Cooking time: 45 minutes

Servings: 8

Ingredients:

1¾ cups homemade vegetable broth

1 cup quinoa, rinsed

Sea salt, to taste

1½ cups cooked chickpeas

1 medium green bell pepper, seeded and chopped

1 medium red bell pepper, seeded and chopped

2 cucumbers, chopped

½ cup scallion (green part only), chopped

1 tablespoon olive oil

2 tablespoons fresh cilantro leaves, chopped

Directions:

1. In a pan, add the broth and bring to a boil over high heat.

2. Add the quinoa and salt and cook until boiling again.

3. Reduce the heat to low and simmer covered for about 15-20 minutes or until all the liquid is absorbed.

4. Remove from the heat and set aside still covered for about 5-10 minutes.

5. Uncover and fluff the quinoa with a fork.

6. In a large serving bowl, add the quinoa and the remaining ingredients and gently toss to coat.

7. Serve immediately.

Nutrition: calories 276, fat 3, carbs 18, protein 28

Conclusion

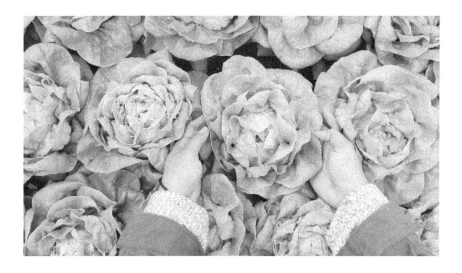

Thank you for making it to the end of the **Dr. Sebi Diet Recipes** book. 'Health is wealth,' many will say, but still, they neglect the call to give proper attention to their health for numerous reasons. Top of the list mostly is the lack of time, but when we are struck by sickness, time eventually pauses because we cannot do what we want. We fail to understand that illnesses and diseases accumulate over time, they do not just appear from nowhere. Your body must have been giving you signs, but you ignored them all.

When you start feeling tired easily, experiencing digestive distress, your allergies become more frequent, you start feeling unhealthy despite eating well, feel weak in your joints, not mentally sharp as usual, and you feel stressed out easily, etc., that is your body sending you a message. This can be likened to a car before it breaks down. It always gives off signals, like starting after several attempts, jerking, and making some weird sounds. These signals are your defense mechanism reacting to the anomalies or impending danger posed by pathogens. So, when we get these signals, we ought to act almost immediately to ensure that our body system gets back to normal.

Most times, the simple thing to do is detox, which is to rid our system of unwanted materials.

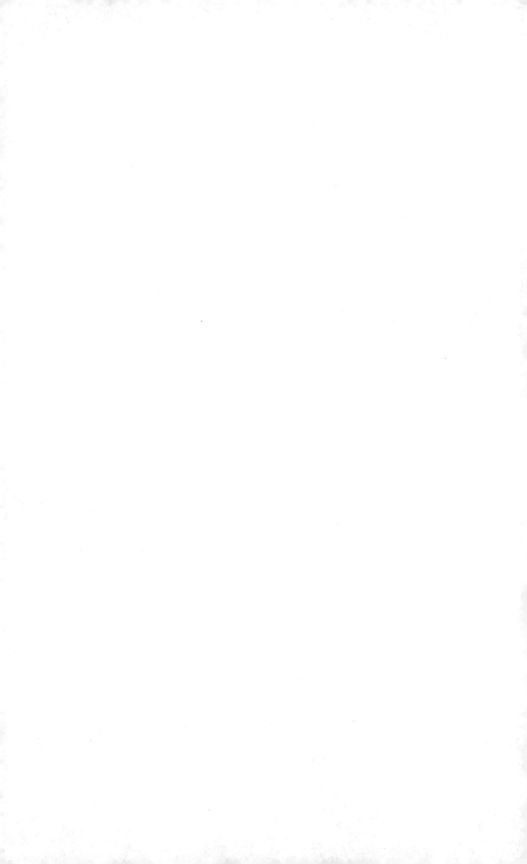

CPSIA information can be obtained
at www.ICGtesting.com
Printed in the USA
BVHW082322030521
606340BV00008B/2289